The Complete Anti-Inflammatory Meat Cookbook

Beef and Chicken Recipes to Fight
Inflammation living a Healthier life

Natalie Worley

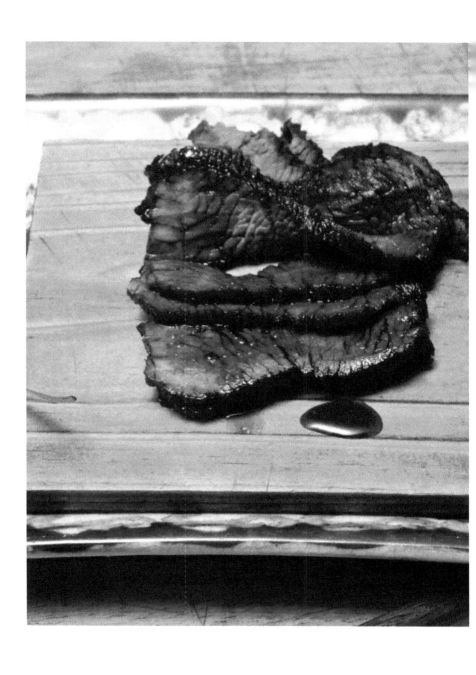

Table of Contents

Chives Turmeric Beef

Prep Time: 10 min | **Cook Time:** 5 hours | **Serve:** 4

- 1 pound beef chops

- 2 teaspoons avocado oil

- 1 teaspoon turmeric powder

- ½ teaspoon sweet paprika

- 1 cup beef stock

- 1 red onion, sliced

- 1 tablespoon chives, chopped

1.In your slow cooker, mix the beef chops with the oil, turmeric, and the other ingredients, toss, put the lid on and cook on High for 5 hours.

2.Divide everything between plates and serve.

Nutrition: 486 calories,38.8g protein, 15.5g carbohydrates, 29.6g fat, 3g fiber, 54mg cholesterol, 204mg sodium, 779mg potassium.

Chili and Garlic Beef

- 1 pound beef chops

- 2 teaspoons avocado oil

- 2 scallions, chopped

- 1 green chili pepper, minced

- ½ teaspoon turmeric powder

- 1 teaspoon chili powder

- ½ cup vegetable stock

- 2 garlic cloves, minced

1.In your slow cooker, mix the beef chops with the oil, scallions, and the other ingredients, toss, put the lid on and cook on High for 4 hours.

2.Divide everything between plates and serve.

Nutrition: 310 calories,23.3g protein, 2.8g

carbohydrates, 21.8g fat, 0.9g fiber, 60mg cholesterol,

470mg sodium, 89mg potassium.

Beef Mix with Onions

Prep Time: 10 min | **Cook Time:** 7 hours | **Serve:** 4

- 1 pound beef loin, cubed

- 2 teaspoons olive oil

- 2 red onions, sliced

- 1 cup Greek-style yogurt

- ¼ cup beef stock

- 1 teaspoon chili powder

- ½ teaspoon rosemary, dried

- 1 tablespoon parsley, chopped

1.In your slow cooker, mix the beef with the onions, oil, and the other ingredients, toss, put the lid on and cook on low for 7 hours.

2.Divide everything between plates and serve.

Nutrition: 252 calories,31.2g protein, 5.7g carbohydrates, 12g fat, 1.5g fiber, 81mg cholesterol, 121mg sodium, 493mg potassium.

Beef and Okra Saute

Prep Time: 10 min | **Cook Time:** 6 hours | **Serve:** 4

- 1 pound beef loin, cubed

- 1 cup okra, sliced

- 2 teaspoons olive oil

- 1 red onion, chopped

- ¼ cup beef stock

- ½ teaspoon chili powder

- ½ teaspoon turmeric powder

- 1 cup tomato passata

1.In your slow cooker, combine the beef with the okra, oil, and the other ingredients, toss, put the lid on and cook on High for 6 hours.

2.Divide the mix between plates and serve.

Nutrition: 258 calories,31.7g protein, 6.4g

carbohydrates, 12g fat, 1.6g fiber, 81mg cholesterol,

118mg sodium, 522mg potassium.

Chives Beef with Cumin

Prep Time: 10 min | **Cook Time:** 4 hours | **Serve:** 4

- 1 pound beef chops
- ½ cup chives, chopped
- ½ cup tomato passata
- 2 scallions, chopped
- 2 teaspoons olive oil
- 2 garlic cloves, minced
- ½ teaspoon sweet paprika
- 1 teaspoon cumin, ground

1.In your slow cooker, mix the beef chops with the chives, passata, and the other ingredients, toss, put the lid on and cook on High for 4 hours,

2.Divide the mix between plates and serve.

Nutrition: 334 calories,22.8g protein, 2.5g carbohydrates, 25.6g fat, 0.5g fiber, 85mg cholesterol, 58mg sodium, 60mg potassium.

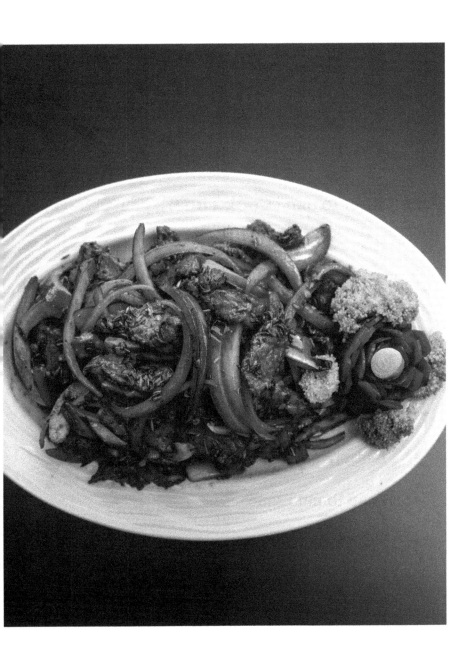

Oregano Beef with Tomato Sauce

Prep Time: 10 min | **Cook Time:** 4 hours | **Serve:** 4

- 1 pound beef loin, cubed
- 1 tablespoon olive oil
- 1 tablespoon balsamic vinegar
- ½ tablespoon lemon juice
- 1 tablespoon oregano, chopped
- ½ cup tomato sauce
- 1 red onion, chopped
- ½ teaspoon chili powder

1.In your slow cooker, mix the beef with the oil, vinegar,

lemon juice, and the other ingredients, toss, put the lid

on and cook on High for 4 hours.

2.Divide the mix between plates and serve right away.

Nutrition: 260 calories,31.2g protein, 5.2g

carbohydrates, 13.3g fat, 1.7g fiber, 81mg cholesterol,

228mg sodium, 557mg potassium.

Beef and Green Beans Bowls

Prep Time: 10 min | **Cook Time:** 6 hours | **Serve:** 4

- 1 pound beef loin, cubed

- 1 tablespoon balsamic vinegar

- 1 cup green beans, trimmed and halved

- 1 tablespoon lime juice

- 1 tablespoon avocado oil

- ½ teaspoon rosemary, dried

- 1 cup beef stock

- 1 tablespoon chives, chopped

1.In your slow cooker, mix the beef loin with the green beans, vinegar, and the other ingredients, toss, put the lid on, and cook on Low for 6 hours.

2.Divide the mix between plates and serve.

Nutrition: 225 calories,31.6g protein, 2.3g

carbohydrates, 10.1g fat, 1.2g fiber, 81mg cholesterol,

230mg sodium, 493mg potassium.

Mint Meat Chops

Prep Time: 10 min | **Cook Time:** 4 hours | **Serve:** 5

- 2 tablespoons olive oil

- 1 pound beef chops

- 1 tablespoon mint, chopped

- ½ teaspoon garam masala

- ½ cup coconut cream

- 1 red onion, chopped

- 2 tablespoons garlic, minced

1.In your slow cooker, mix the beef chops with the oil, mint, and the other ingredients, toss, put the lid on and cook on High for 4 hours.

2.Divide the mix between plates and serve warm.

Nutrition: 360 calories,19g protein, 4.6g carbohydrates, 29.9g fat, 1.2g fiber, 68mg cholesterol, 128mg sodium, 127mg potassium.

Beef and Vegetable Plates

Prep Time: 10 min | **Cook Time:** 7 hours | **Serve:** 4

- 1 tablespoon avocado oil

- 1 pound beef loin, cubed

- 2 scallions, chopped

- 1 cup artichoke hearts

- ½ teaspoon chili powder

- 1 cup tomato passata

- ¼ tablespoon dill, chopped

1.In your slow cooker, combine the beef with the artichokes and the other ingredients, toss, put the lid on and cook on Low for 7 hours.

2.Divide the mix between plates and serve.

Nutrition: 230 calories,31.2g protein, 4.4g carbohydrates, 10g fat, 1g fiber, 81mg cholesterol, 167mg sodium, 430mg potassium.

Beef with Paprika and Sweet Potato

Prep Time: 10 min | **Cook Time:** 4 hours | **Serve:** 4

- 1 pound beef loin, roughly cubed

- 2 sweet potatoes, peeled and cubed

- ½ cup beef stock

- ½ cup tomato sauce

- ½ teaspoon sweet paprika

- ½ teaspoon coriander, ground

- 1 tablespoon avocado oil

- 1 tablespoon balsamic vinegar

- 1 tablespoon cilantro, chopped

1.In your slow cooker, mix the beef with the potatoes, stock, sauce, and the other ingredients toss, put the lid on and cook on High for 4 hours

2.Divide everything between plates and serve.

Nutrition: 266 calories,31.7g protein, 12.5g carbohydrates, 10.1g fat, 2.3g fiber, 81mg cholesterol, 324mg sodium, 829mg potassium.

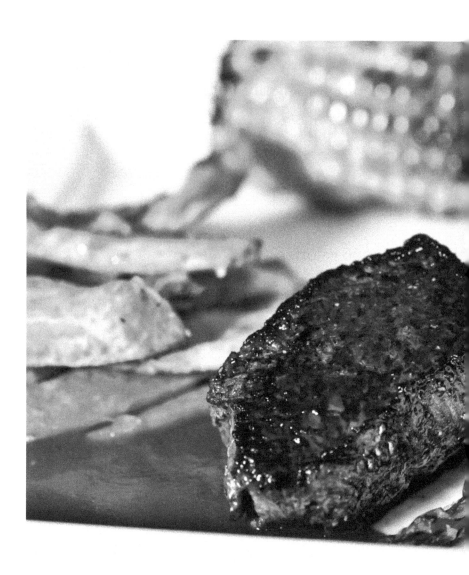

Oregano and Basil Beef

Prep Time: 10 min | **Cook Time:** 4 hours | **Serve:** 4

- 1 teaspoon olive oil

- 1 pound beef loin, cubed

- 1 cup cherry tomatoes, halved

- 1 tablespoon basil, chopped

- ½ teaspoon rosemary, dried

- 1 tablespoon oregano, chopped

- 1 cup beef stock

- ½ teaspoon sweet paprika

- 1 tablespoon parsley, chopped

1.Grease the slow cooker with the oil and mix the beef with the tomatoes, basil, and the other ingredients inside.

2.Toss, put the lid on, cook on High for 4 hours, divide the mix between plates and serve.

Nutrition: 234 calories,31.6g protein, 2.8g carbohydrates, 11g fat, 1.2g fiber, 81mg cholesterol, 261mg sodium, 558mg potassium.

Tender Beef with Eggplants

Prep Time: 10 min | **Cook Time:** 7 hours | **Serve:** 4

- 1 pound beef loin, cubed

- 1 eggplant, cubed

- 2 scallions, chopped

- 2 garlic cloves, minced

- ½ cup beef stock

- ¼ cup tomato sauce

- 1 teaspoon sweet paprika

- 1 tablespoon chives, chopped

1.In your slow cooker, mix the beef loin with the scallions, eggplant, and the other ingredients, toss, put the lid on and cook on Low for 7 hours.

2.Divide the mix between plates and serve right away.

Nutrition: 247 calories,32.3g protein, 8.9g

carbohydrates, 9.9g fat, 4.7g fiber, 81mg cholesterol,

244mg sodium, 756mg potassium.

Lemon Beef with Onions

Prep Time: 10 min | **Cook Time:** 7 hours | **Serve:** 4

- 1 pound beef loin, cubed

- 1 red onion, sliced

- ½ cup tomato sauce

- 1 tablespoon balsamic vinegar

- 1 tablespoon lemon juice

- 1 tablespoon lemon zest, grated

- 1 teaspoon olive oil

- 3 garlic cloves, chopped

- 1 tablespoon chives, chopped

1.In your slow cooker, mix the beef with the onion, tomato sauce, and the other ingredients, toss, put the lid on, and cook on Low for 7 hours.

2Divide the mix between plates and serve right away.

Nutrition: 241 calories,31.3g protein, 5.4g

carbohydrates, 10.8g fat, 1.2g fiber, 81mg cholesterol,

225mg sodium, 550mg potassium.

Rosemary Beef with Scallions

- 1 pound beef chops

- 1 tablespoon olive oil

- 3 garlic cloves, minced

- 1 tablespoon rosemary, chopped

- 1 cup kalamata olives, pitted and halved

- 3 scallions, chopped

- 1 teaspoon turmeric powder

- 1 cup beef stock

1.In your slow cooker, mix the beef chops with the oil, rosemary, and the other ingredients, toss, put the lid on and cook on High for 4 hours.

2.Divide the mix between plates and serve.

Nutrition: 386 calories,23.5g protein, 4.6g

carbohydrates, 30.5g fat, 1.9g fiber, 85mg cholesterol,

547mg sodium, 97mg potassium.

Nutmeg Beef

Prep Time: 10 min | **Cook Time:** 6 hours | **Serve:** 4

- 1 pound beef loin, roughly cubed
- 1 cup butternut squash, peeled and cubed ½ teaspoon nutmeg, ground ½ teaspoon chili powder
- ½ teaspoon coriander, ground
- 2 teaspoons olive oil
- 1 cup beef stock
- 1 tablespoon cilantro, chopped

1.In your slow cooker, mix the beef with the squash, nutmeg, and the other ingredients, toss, put the lid on and cook on Low for 6 hours.

2.Divide the mix between plates and serve.

Nutrition: 249 calories,31.4g protein, 4.4g carbohydrates, 12.1g fat, 0.9g fiber, 81mg cholesterol, 263mg sodium, 549mg potassium.

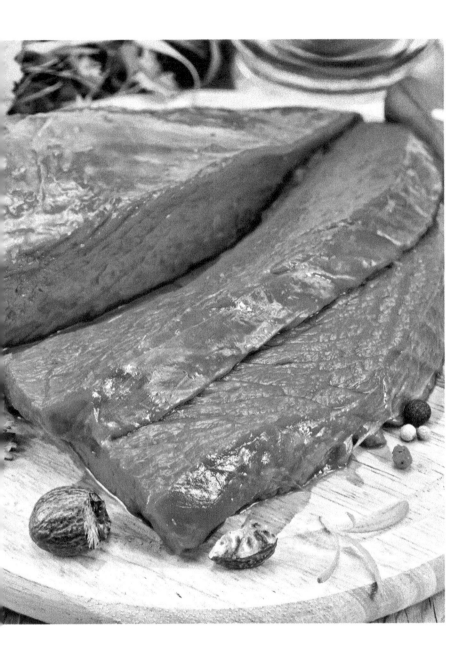

Aromatic Fennel Beef

Prep Time: 10 min | **Cook Time:** 4 hours | **Serve:** 4

- 1 pound beef loin, roughly cubed

- 1 fennel bulb, sliced

- 1 tablespoon lemon juice

- 1 teaspoon avocado oil

- ½ teaspoon coriander, ground

- 1 cup tomato passata

- 1 tablespoon cilantro, chopped

1.In your slow cooker, combine the beef with the fennel, lemon juice, and the other ingredients, toss, put the lid on and cook on High for 4 hours.

2.Divide the mix between plates and serve.

Nutrition: 235 calories,31.5g protein, 6g carbohydrates, 9.8g fat, 1.9g fiber, 81mg cholesterol, 94mg sodium, 636mg potassium.

Creamy Beef with Turmeric

Prep Time: 10 min | **Cook Time:** 6 hours | **Serve:** 4

- 2 pounds beef loin, cubed
- 1 cup Greek-style yogurt
- 1/3 cup beef stock
- 2 teaspoons avocado oil
- 1 teaspoon turmeric powder
- 1 red onion, sliced
- 1 tablespoon cilantro, chopped

1.In your slow cooker, mix the beef with the stock, oil, and the other ingredients except for the greek style yogurt, toss, put the lid on, and cook on Low for 5 hours.

2.Add the cream, toss, cook on Low for 1 more hour, divide the mix into bowls and serve.

Nutrition: 470 calories,67g protein, 5.4g carbohydrates, 20.1g fat, 0.8g fiber, 166mg cholesterol, 216mg sodium, 918mg potassium.

Beef with Capers

Prep Time: 10 min | **Cook Time:** 7 hours | **Serve:** 4

- 1 pound beef loin, cubed

- 1 tablespoon capers, drained

- 1 cup greek style yogurt

- ½ cup beef stock

- ½ tablespoon mustard

- 3 scallions, chopped

- 2 teaspoons avocado oil

- 1 teaspoon cumin, ground

- 1 tablespoon parsley, chopped

1.In your slow cooker, mix the beef with capers, stock, and the other ingredients except for the yogurt, toss, put the lid on, and cook on Low for 6 hours.

2.Add the yogurt, toss, cook on Low for 1 more hour,

divide the mix between plates and serve.

Nutrition: 258 calories,32.4g protein, 4.9g

carbohydrates, 12.3g fat, 0.8g fiber, 81mg cholesterol,

237mg sodium, 460mg potassium.

Masala Beef

Prep Time: 10 min | **Cook Time:** 7 hours | **Serve:** 4

- 1 pound beef loin, cubed

- 1 teaspoon garam masala

- 1 tablespoon olive oil

- 1 tablespoon lime zest, grated

- 1 tablespoon lime juice

- ½ teaspoon sweet paprika

- ½ teaspoon coriander, ground

- 1 cup beef stock

1.In your slow cooker, mix the beef with the garam masala, oil, and the other ingredients, toss, put the lid on and cook on Low for 7 hours.

2.Divide the mix between plates and serve.

Nutrition: 244 calories,31.1g protein, 0.9g

carbohydrates, 13.1g fat, 0.3g fiber, 81mg cholesterol,

260mg sodium, 432mg potassium.

Cabbage and Beef Saute

Prep Time: 10 min | **Cook Time:** 5 hours | **Serve:** 8

- 2 pounds beef loin, cubed

- 1 cup red cabbage, shredded

- 1 cup beef stock

- 1 teaspoon avocado oil

- 1 teaspoon sweet paprika

- 2 tablespoons tomato paste

- 1 tablespoon cilantro, chopped

1.In your slow cooker, mix the beef with the cabbage, stock, and the other ingredients, toss, put the lid on and cook on High for 5 hours.

2.Divide everything between plates and serve.

Nutrition: 216 calories,31g protein, 1.5g carbohydrates,

9.7g fat, 0.5g fiber, 81mg cholesterol, 166mg sodium,

466mg potassium.

Tender Beef with Lentils

Prep Time: 10 min | **Cook Time:** 7 hours | **Serve:** 4

- 1 pound beef loin, cubed

- 1 cup lentils, drained and rinsed, cooked

- 1 tablespoon olive oil

- 1 yellow onion, chopped

- ¼ cup tomato sauce

- ¼ cup beef stock

- 1 tablespoon cilantro, chopped

1.In your slow cooker, mix the beef with the lentils, oil, onion, and the other ingredients, toss, put the lid on and cook on Low for 7 hours.

2.Divide the mix between plates and serve.

Nutrition: 423 calories,44.3g protein, 32.3g carbohydrates, 13.6g fat, 15.5g fiber, 81mg cholesterol, 196mg sodium, 944mg potassium.

Coriander Beef Mix

Prep Time: 10 min | **Cook Time:** 7 hours | **Serve:** 4

- 1 pound beef loin, cubed
- 2 teaspoons avocado oil
- 1 tablespoon balsamic vinegar
- ½ teaspoon coriander, ground
- 1 cup beef stock

1.In your slow cooker, mix the beef with the oil, vinegar, and the other ingredients, toss, put the lid on and cook on Low for 7 hours.

2.Divide the mix between plates and serve with a side salad.

Nutrition: 214 calories,31g protein, 0.2g carbohydrates, 9.9g fat, 0.1g fiber, 81mg cholesterol, 258mg sodium, 428mg potassium.

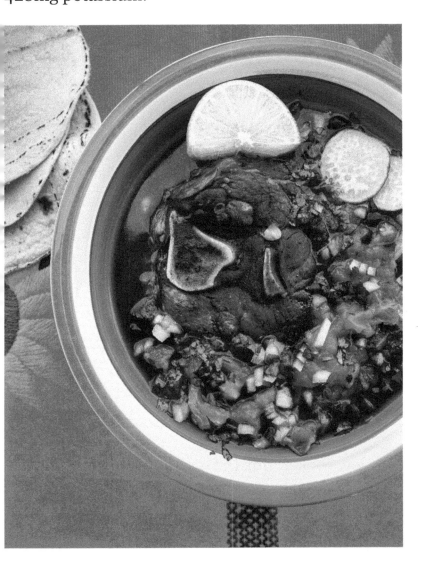

Beef and Endives Bowls

Prep Time: 10 min | **Cook Time:** 7 hours | **Serve:** 4

- 1 pound beef loin, cubed

- 2 teaspoons avocado oil

- 2 endives, shredded

- ½ cup beef stock

- ½ teaspoon sweet paprika

- ¼ cup tomato passata

- 3 garlic cloves, minced

- 1 tablespoon chives, chopped

1.In your slow cooker, mix the meat with the oil, endives, and the other ingredients, toss, put the lid on and cook on Low for 7 hours.

2.Divide the mix between plates and serve.

Nutrition: 261 calories,34.2g protein, 10g carbohydrates, 10.4g fat, 8.2g fiber, 81mg cholesterol, 217mg sodium, 1232mg potassium.

Beef and Lime

Prep Time: 10 min | **Cook Time:** 4 hours | **Serve:** 4

- 1 pound beef loin, roughly cubed

- 2 small zucchinis, cubed

- Juice of 1 lime

- ½ teaspoon rosemary, dried

- 2 tablespoons avocado oil

- 1 red onion, chopped

- ½ cup beef stock

- 1 tablespoon garlic, minced

- 1 tablespoon cilantro, chopped

1.In your slow cooker, mix the beef with the zucchinis, lime juice, and the other ingredients, toss, put the lid on and cook on High for 4 hours.

2.Divide the mix between plates and serve.

Nutrition: 242 calories,31.9g protein, 5.8g
carbohydrates, 10.6g fat, 1.7g fiber, 81mg cholesterol,
168mg sodium, 630mg potassium.

Beef Curry with Mustard

Prep Time: 10 min | **Cook Time:** 8 hours | **Serve:** 8

- 2 pounds beef steak, cubed

- 2 tablespoons olive oil

- 3 potatoes, diced

- 1 tablespoon mustard

- 2 ½ tablespoons curry powder

- 2 yellow onions, chopped

- 2 garlic cloves, minced

- 10 ounces of coconut milk

- 2 tablespoons tomato sauce

1.In your Slow cooker, mix oil with steak, potatoes,

mustard, curry powder, garlic, coconut milk, tomato

sauce, pepper, toss, cover, and cook on Low for 8 hours.

2.Stir curry one more time, divide into bowls and serve.

Nutrition: 403 calories,37.6g protein, 19.2g

carbohydrates, 19.8g fat, 4.2g fiber, 101mg cholesterol,

107mg 971mg sodium, potassium.

Herby Chicken Fillets

Prep Time: 15 minutes | **Serve:** 6

- 1 1/2 pounds chicken fillets

- 1 1/2 tablespoons olive oil

- 1/2 teaspoon ground black pepper

- 1 teaspoon kosher salt

- 1 stick butter

- 2 teaspoons apple cider vinegar

- 1/3 cup chopped fresh cilantro

- 2 tablespoons finely minced shallots

- 1 teaspoon finely minced garlic

1.Preheat a skillet over moderate heat. Add the olive oil.

Fry the chicken fillets for around 10 minutes until they

are brown.

2.In a bowl mix together the salt, pepper, butter, apple

cider vinegar, cilantro, shallots and garlic.

3.Serve the chicken fillets with the herby sauce.

Nutrition: Calories 258.6, Protein 15.2g, Fat 20.2g

Carbs 4g Sugar 1.5g

Turkey Meatballs with a side of Basil Chutney

Prep Time: 30 minutes | **Serve:** 6

For the Meatballs:

- 2 tablespoons olive oil

- 1 1/2 pounds ground turkey

- 1/4 teaspoon ground black pepper

- 1/2 teaspoon sea salt

- ½ teaspoon celery seeds 1/4 teaspoon dried thyme 1/2 teaspoon onion powder 1/2 teaspoon garlic powder

- 3 tablespoons flax seed meal 1/2 teaspoons paprika

- ½ cup grated Parmesan cheese

-

- 2 small-sized eggs, lightly beaten

For the Basil Chutney:

- 1/2 cup fresh basil leaves

- 1/2 cup coriander leaves

- 2 tablespoons fresh lemon juice

- 1 teaspoon grated fresh ginger root

- 2 tablespoons water

- 2 tablespoons olive oil

- Salt and pepper, to taste

- 1 tablespoon minced green chili

1.Mix all the meatball ingredients. Form into 16 balls and put to one side.

2.Preheat a skillet over medium heat and then heat the olive oil. Fry the meatballs for 7 -8 minutes, making sure that all sides are browned.

3.Then make the chutney. Put the basil leaves, coriander leaves, lemon juice, ginger, olive oil, salt, pepper and chil into a food processor and blend.

Nutrition: Calories 260, Protein 25.4g, Fat 15g, Carbs 6g, Sugar 2.1g

Asian Saucy Chicken

Prep Time: 25 minutes | **Serve:** 4

- 1 tablespoon sesame oil

- 4 chicken legs

- 1/4 cup Shaoxing wine

- 2 tablespoons brown erythritol

- 1/4 cup spicy tomato sauce

1.Heat the sesame oil in a wok over medium-high heat.

Fry the chicken until golden in color; reserve.

2.Add Shaoxing wine to deglaze the pan.

3.Add in erythritol and spicy tomato sauce, and bring the

mixture to a boil.

4.Then, immediately reduce the heat to medium-low.

5.Let it simmer for about 10 minutes until the sauce coats

the back of a spoon.

6.Add the chicken back to the wok.

7.Continue to cook until the chicken is sticky and golden

or about 4 minutes.

Nutrition: 367 Calories; 14.7g Fat; 3.5g Carbs; 51.2g

Protein; 1.1g Fiber

Duck Stew Olla Tapada

Prep Time: 30 minutes | **Serve:** 3

- 1 red bell pepper, deveined and chopped

- 1 pound duck breasts, boneless, skinless, and chopped into small chunks

- 1/2 cup chayote, peeled and cubed

- 1 shallot, chopped

- 1 teaspoon Mexican spice mix

1.In a clay pot, heat 2 teaspoons of canola oil over a medium-high flame. Sauté the peppers and shallot until softened about 4 minutes.

2.Add in the remaining ingredients; pour in 1 ½ cups of water or chicken bone broth. Once your mixture starts boiling, reduce the heat to medium-low.

3.Let it simmer, partially covered, for 18 to 22 minutes, until cooked through.

Nutrition: 228 Calories; 9.5g Fat; 3.3g Carbs; 30.6g Protein; 1g Fiber

Cheesy Ranch Chicken

Prep Time: 20 minutes | **Serve:** 4

- 2 chicken breasts

- 1/2 tablespoon ranch seasoning mix

- 4 slices bacon, chopped

- 1/2 cup Monterey-Jack cheese, grated

- 4 ounces Ricotta cheese, room temperature

1.Preheat your oven to 360 degrees F.

2.Rub the chicken with ranch seasoning mix.

3.Heat a saucepan over medium-high flame. Now, sear the chicken for about 8 minutes. Lower the chicken into a lightly greased casserole dish.

4.Top with cheese and bacon and bake in the preheated oven for about 10 minutes until hot and bubbly. Serve with freshly snipped scallions, if desired.

Nutrition: 295 Calories; 19.5g Fat; 2.9g Carbs; 25.5g Protein; 0.4g Fiber

Turkey Crust Meatza

Prep Time: 35 minutes | **Serve:** 4

- ½ pound ground turkey

- 2 slices Canadian bacon

- 1 tomato, chopped

- 1 tablespoon pizza spice mix

- 1 cup Mozzarella cheese, grated

1.Mix the ground turkey and cheese; season with salt and black pepper and mix until everything is well combined.

2.Press the mixture into a foil-lined baking pan. Bake in the preheated oven at 380 degrees F for 25 minutes.

3.Top the crust with Canadian bacon, tomato, and pizza spice mix. Continue to bake for a further 8 minutes.

4.Let it rest a couple of minutes before slicing and.

Nutrition: 360 Calories; 22.7g Fat; 5.9g Carbs; 32.6g Protein; 0.7g Fiber

Simple Turkey Goulash

Prep Time: 45 minutes | **Serve:** 6

- 2 tablespoons olive oil

- 1 large-sized leek, chopped

- 2 cloves garlic, minced

- 2 pounds turkey thighs, skinless, boneless and chopped

- 2 celery stalks, chopped

1.In a clay pot, heat 2 olive oil over a medium-high flame. Then, cook the leeks until tender and translucent.

2.Then, continue to sauté the garlic for 30 seconds to 1 minute.

3.Stir in the turkey, celery, and 4 cups of water. Once your mixture starts boiling, let it simmer, partially covered, for about 40 minutes.

Nutrition: 220 Calories; 7.4g Fat; 2.7g Carbs; 35.5g Protein; 1g Fiber

Fajita with Zucchini

Prep Time: 20 minutes | **Serve:** 4

- 1 red onion, sliced

- 1 teaspoon Fajita seasoning mix

- 1 pound turkey cutlets

- 1 zucchini, spiralized

- 1 chili pepper, chopped

1.In a nonstick skillet, heat 1 tablespoon of the olive oil over a medium-high flame. Cook the turkey cutlets for 6 to 7 minutes on each side. Slice the meat into strips and reserve.

2.Heat another tablespoon of olive oil and sauté the onion and chili pepper until they are just tender. Sprinkle with Fajita seasoning mix.

3.Add in the zucchini and the reserved turkey; let it cook

for 4 minutes more or until everything is cooked through

Serve with 1/2 cup of salsa, if desired. Enjoy!

Nutrition: 212 Calories; 9.2g Fat; 5.6g Carbs; 26g

Protein; 1.2g Fiber

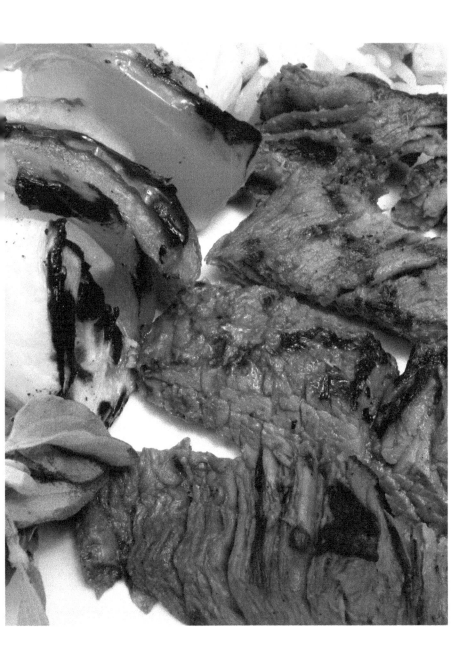

Easiest Turkey Meatballs Ever

Prep Time: 1 hour 20 minutes | **Serve:** 4

- 1 egg, whisked

- 4 spring onions, finely chopped

- 1/2 cup parmesan cheese, grated

- 1 tablespoon Italian spice mix

- 1 pound ground turkey

1.Thoroughly combine all ingredients. Roll the turkey

mixture into balls and place them in your refrigerator for

1 hour.

2.In a cast-iron skillet, heat 2 tablespoons of olive oil

over medium-high heat.

3.Sear the meatballs for 12 minutes or until nicely

browned on all sides.

Nutrition: 366 Calories; 27.7g Fat; 3g Carbs; 25.9g Protein; 0.5g Fiber

Greek-Style Chicken Drumet

Prep Time: 30 minutes | **Serve:** 2

- 1 tablespoon olive oil

- 6 Kalamata olives, pitted and sliced

- 1 pound chicken drumettes

- 6 ounces tomato sauce

- 1 teaspoon Greek seasoning blend

1.Rub the chicken drumettes with Greek seasoning blend.

2.In a nonstick skillet, heat the olive oil over medium-high flame. Sear the chicken for about 10 minutes until nicely brown.

3.Add in the olives and tomato sauce. Stir and continue to cook, partially covered, for about 18 minutes until everything is thoroughly heated. Bon appétit!

Nutrition: 341 Calories; 14.3g Fat; 3.6g Carbs; 47g Protein; 1.1g Fiber

Chicken Tawook Salad

Prep Time: 20 minutes | **Serve:** 2

- 2 chicken breasts

- 4 tablespoons apple cider vinegar

- 1 cup grape tomatoes, halved

- 1 Lebanese cucumber, thinly sliced

- 2 tablespoons extra-virgin olive oil

1.Preheat a grill to medium-high and oil a grill grate. Gril the chicken for about 13 minutes, turing them over a few times.

2.Slice the chicken into the bite-sized chunks and transfer them to a bowl. Add in the vinegar, tomatoes, cucumber, and olive oil. Toss to combine well.

Nutrition: 403 Calories; 18g Fat; 5.3g Carbs; 51.6g

Protein; 1.6g Fiber

Greek Chicken with Peppers

Prep Time: 20 minutes | **Serve:** 2

- 2 chicken drumsticks, boneless and skinless

- 2 bell peppers, deveined and halved

- 1 small chili pepper, finely chopped

- 2 tablespoons Greek aioli

- 6 Kalamata olives, pitted

1.Rub the chicken with 1 tablespoon of extra-virgin olive oil. Season with salt and black pepper to taste.

2.Grill the chicken drumsticks for 8 to 9 minutes; add the bell peppers and grill them for a further 6 minutes.

3.Place the meat and peppers in a bowl; add in chili pepper and Greek aioli.

4.Top with Kalamata olives and serve.

Nutrition: 403 Calories; 31.4g Fat; 5g Carbs; 24.5g

Protein; 1.1g Fiber

Colorful Chicken Chowder

Prep Time: 50 minutes | **Serve:** 6

- 1 tablespoon olive oil

- 6 chicken wings

- 1 cup mixed frozen vegetables (celery, onions, and pepper

- 1 tablespoon poultry seasoning mix

- 1 whole egg

1.Heat the olive oil in a heavy-bottomed pot over medium-high heat. Then, brown the chicken for 10 minutes or until no longer pink; set them aside.

2.Then, cook the vegetables in the pan drippings until they are crisp-tender.

3.Season with poultry seasoning mix and turn the heat to medium-low; continue to simmer for a further 40 minutes or until everything is thoroughly cooked.

4.Chop the chicken and discard the fat and bones.

5.Whisk the egg into the cooking liquid. Add the reserved chicken back to the pot. Taste and adjust the seasonings.

Nutrition: 283 Calories; 18.9g Fat; 2.6g Carbs; 25.4g Protein; 0.5g Fiber

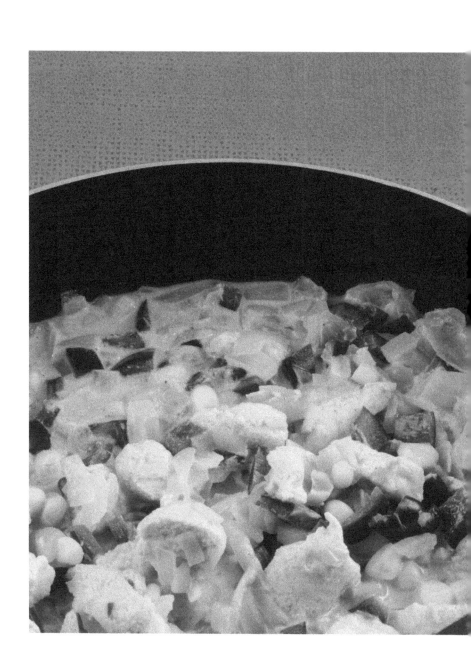

Chicken Frittata with Asiago

Cheese and Herbs

Prep Time: 30 minutes | **Serve:** 4

- 1-pound chicken breasts, cut into small strips

- 4 slices of bacon

- 1 cup Asiago cheese, shredded

- 6 eggs

- 1/2 cup yogurt

1.Preheat an oven-proof skillet. Then, fry the bacon until crisp and reserve. Then, cook the chicken for about 8 minutes or until no longer pink in the pan drippings.

2.Add the reserved bacon back to the skillet.

3.In a mixing dish, thoroughly combine the eggs and yogurt; season with Italian spice mix.

4.Pour the egg mixture over the chicken and bacon. Top with cheese and bake in the preheated oven at 380 degrees F for 22 minutes until hot and bubbly.

5.Let it rest a couple of minutes before slicing.

Nutrition: 484 Calories; 31.8g Fat; 5.8g Carbs; 41.9g Protein; 0.7g Fiber

Stuffed Chicken with Sauerkraut and Cheese

Prep Time: 35 minutes | **Serve:** 5

- 5 chicken cutlets

- 1 cup Romano cheese, shredded

- 2 garlic cloves, minced

- 5 Italian peppers, deveined and chopped

- 5 tablespoons sauerkraut

1.Spritz a baking pan with 1 tablespoon of the olive oil.

Brush the chicken with another tablespoon of olive oil.

2.Season the chicken with Italian spice mix. You can

spread Dijon mustard on one side of each chicken cutlet,

if desired.

3.Divide the garlic, peppers and Romano cheese between chicken cutlets; roll them up.

4.Bake at 360 degrees F for 25 to 33 minutes until nicely brown on all sides. Serve with the sauerkraut and serve.

Nutrition: 376 Calories; 16.7g Fat; 5.8g Carbs; 47g Protein; 1g Fiber

Cream of Chicken Soup

- 1/2 cup Italian peppers, deseeded and chopped
- 1/2 cup green cabbage, shredded
- 5 chicken thighs
- 1/2 cup celery, chopped
- 7 ounces full-fat cream cheese

1.Add Italian peppers, cabbage, chicken thighs, and celery to a large clay pot.

2.Pour in 5 cups of water or chicken broth.

3.Partially cover and let it simmer over medium-high heat approximately 30 minutes. Transfer the chicken to a cutting board,

4.Shred the chicken and return it to the pot. Add in full-fat cream cheese and stir until everything is well incorporated.

Nutrition: 514 Calories; 38g Fat; 5.4g Carbs; 35.3g Protein; 0.5g Fiber

Lemony and Garlicky Chicken Wings

Prep Time: 25 minutes + marinating time | **Serve:** 4

- 8 chicken wings
- 2 garlic cloves, minced
- 1/4 cup leeks, chopped
- 2 tablespoons lemon juice
- 1 teaspoon Mediterranean spice mix

1.Place all ingredients in a ceramic dish. Cover and let it sit in your refrigerator for 2 hours.

2.Brush the chicken wings with melted ghee. Grill the chicken wings for 15 to 20 minutes, turning them occasionally to ensure even cooking.

Nutrition: 131 Calories; 7.8g Fat; 1.8g Carbs; 13.4g

Protein; 0.3g Fiber

Creamiest Chicken Salad Ever

Prep Time: 1 hour 20 minutes | **Serve:** 3

- 1 chicken breast, skinless

- 1/4 mayonnaise

- 1/4 cup sour cream

- 2 tablespoons Cottage cheese, room temperature

- 1/2 avocado, peeled and cubed

1.Cook the chicken in a pot of salted water. Remove from the heat and let the chicken sit, covered, in the hot water for 10 to 15 minutes.

2.Slice the chicken into bite-sized strips. Toss with the remaining ingredients.

3.Place in the refrigerator for at least one hour. Serve

well chilled.

Nutrition: 400 Calories; 35.1g Fat; 5.6g Carbs; 16.1g

Protein; 1g Fiber

Thai Turkey Curry

Prep Time: 1 hour | **Serve:** 4

- 1 pound turkey wings, boneless and chopped

- 2 cloves garlic, finely chopped

- 1 Thai red chili pepper, minced

- 1 cup unsweetened coconut milk, preferably homemade

- 1 cup turkey consommé

1.In a saucepan, warm 2 teaspoons of sesame oil. Once hot, brown turkey about 8 minutes or until it is golden brown.

2.Add in the garlic and Thai chili pepper and continue to cook for a minute or so.

3.Add coconut milk and consommé. Season with salt and black pepper to taste. Continue to cook for 40 to 45 minutes over medium heat. Serve warm and enjoy!

Nutrition: 295 Calories; 19.5g Fat; 2.9g Carbs; 25.5g Protein; 1g Fiber

Baked Teriyaki Turkey

Prep Time: 15 minutes | **Serve:** 2

- ¾ pound lean ground turkey

- 1 brown onion, chopped

- 1 red bell pepper, deveined and chopped

- 1 serrano pepper, deveined and chopped

- ¼ cup keto teriyaki sauce

1.Cook the ground turkey in the preheated pan over medium-high heat; cook for about 5 minutes until no longer pink.

2.Now, sauté the onion and peppers for 3 minutes more. Add in teriyaki sauce and bring the mixture to a boil.

3.Immediately remove from the heat; add in the cooked ground turkey and sautéed mixture.

Nutrition: 410 Calories; 27.1g Fat; 6.6g Carbs; 36.5g Protein; 1g Fiber

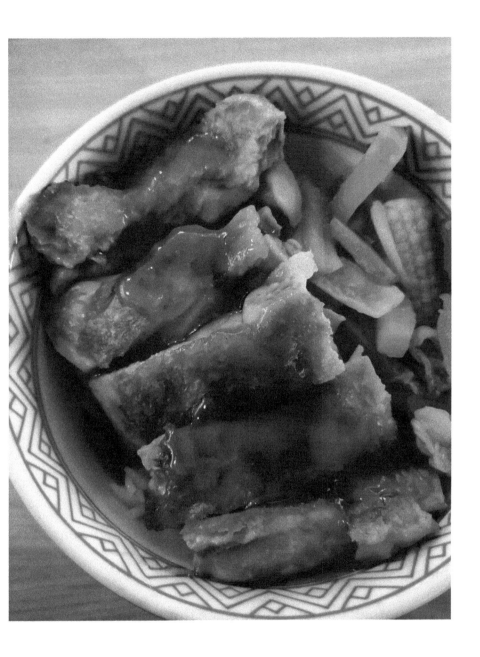

Ranch Turkey with Greek Sauce

Prep Time: 20 minutes | **Serve:** 4

- 2 eggs

- 1 tablespoon Ranch seasoning blend

- ½ cup almond meal

- 1 pound turkey tenders, 1/2-inch thick

- ½ cup Greek keto sauce

1.In a shallow bowl, whisk the eggs with Ranch seasoning blend.

2.In another shallow bowl, place the almond meal. Dip the turkey tenders into the Ranch egg mixture.

3.Then, press them into the almond meal; press to coat well.

4.Heat 2 tablespoons of olive oil in a pan over medium-high heat. Brown turkey tenders for 3 to 4 minutes on each side.

5.Serve the turkey tenders with Greek keto sauce. Enjoy!

Nutrition: 396 Calories; 27.5g Fat; 3.9g Carbs; 33.1g Protein; 1.9g Fiber

Mediterranean Herbed Chicken

Prep Time: 20 minutes | **Serve:** 5

- 2 tablespoons butter, softened at room temperature
- 5 chicken legs, skinless
- 2 scallions, chopped
- 1 tablespoon Mediterranean spice mix
- 1 cup vegetable broth

1.In a saucepan, melt 1 tablespoon of butter over a medium-high flame. Now, brown the chicken legs for about 10 minutes, turning them periodically.

2.Add in the remaining tablespoon of butter, scallions,

Mediterranean spice mix, and broth. When your mixture

reaches boiling, reduce the temperature to a simmer.

3.Continue to simmer for 10 to 11 minutes until cooked

through. Taste and adjust the seasoning. Bon appétit!

Nutrition: 370 Calories; 16g Fat; 0.9g Carbs; 51g

Protein; 0.2g Fiber

Saucy Chicken with Marsala Wine

Prep Time: 20 minutes | **Serve:** 2

- 2 chicken fillets
- 1/4 cup marsala wine
- 1 cup broccoli florets
- 1/4 tomato paste
- 1/2 cup double cream

1.Heat 1 tablespoon of olive oil in a sauté pan over medium-high heat. Once hot, sear the chicken for 10 minutes, flipping them over once or twice.

2.Add marsala wine and deglaze the pot. Add in the broccoli and tomato paste.

3.Reduce the heat to simmer.

4.Continue to simmer for a further 5 to 7 minutes. Lastly, stir in the double cream. Season with paprika, salt, and black pepper to taste.

Nutrition: 347 Calories; 20.4g Fat; 4.7g Carbs; 35.3g Protein; 1.4g Fiber

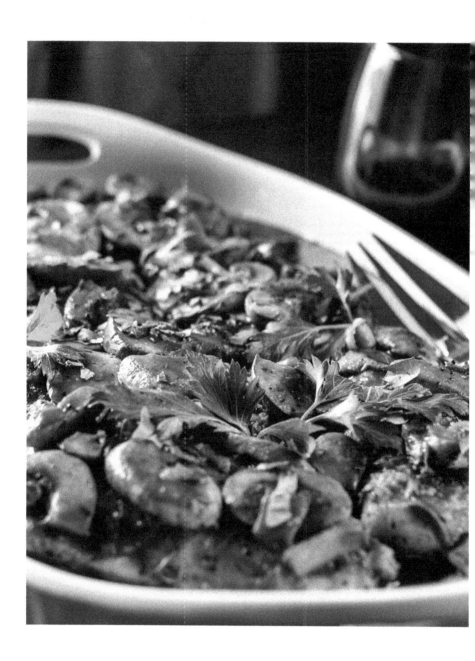

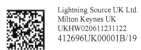

9 781802 773422